My Bingo Pals

ISBN: 1-4663-6200-6
ISBN-13: 9781466362000

My Bingo Pals

Henry Nelson Feste

2011

Acknowledgements

It was my daughter Alyssa's persistence that convinced me to proceed and offer my services at a local health care center. I've been a bingo caller for seniors for almost three years now at this care center. My story is all about my volunteer work with these seniors. Thank you, Alyssa, for your efforts, for without them, I may not have volunteered, and there would be no story.

Thanks also to my wife, Helen, for without her help I doubt that I could have gone on volunteering with as much success as I have had. She is a very organized person, and as such she has kept me on the right path. Many thanks, Helen, for this and for your tireless help.

Thanks also goes out to my son, Billy, a writer himself, for his advice, and to my daughter Linda and son-in-law Jim for their help with the artistry and photography work of this story.

My Bingo Pals

I'm Henry—or Hank, if you prefer. Just about everybody calls me Hank, while my wife, family, and others call me Henry. I've been retired for the past eight years. Being retired means more time with loved ones, hobbies, and other activities, but it often falls short of filling the gap of a lifetime of hard work. My wife, two daughters, and son have all urged me to use what spare time I have to do volunteer work. I thought about it, but that's all—until my daughter Alyssa, who lives nearby, insisted that I respond to a local newspaper ad for bingo volunteers at a local care center. She said that I was suited for this type of volunteer work, having called bingo for my kids and grandkids. And so I responded to the ad and started calling bingo for seniors in April 2009, a senior myself at seventy-five years of age.

My wife and I were witness to the early ground breaking, construction, and final completion of this care center, which is located near our home, in 2007. Little did I or my wife know then that I would be a volunteer at this care center in 2009. Soon after the care center was completed, seniors moved into the new facility, which has a large administrative staff and a full complement of doctors, nurses, nurses' aides, and caregivers that provide IV, physical, occupational, and speech therapy, as well as short/long-term care for the elderly.

Henry Nelson Feste

As I entered this care center for the first time, I could not help but notice the beehive of activity going on, as staff, doctors, nurses, and caregivers scurried about, giving care to seniors, many of them in wheelchairs or requiring walkers, and some requiring intensive care on gurneys or while bedridden. I experienced this as I walked past the building's large covered front porch, crowded with mostly wheelchair-confined seniors, and entered the building by way of large entrance doorways into a large foyer, where I was greeted by a reception- ist. Following her direction, I proceeded to walk down a long, wide hallway that brought me to the center's hub of activity, a very large, somewhat circular room with a cir- cular station of counters at its center housing computers and other equipment. I immediately noticed that behind these counters, doctors and nurses were busy providing medicine and medical care to seniors. I was in awe at the sight of this care going on around me as I walked by on my way to meet with the center's activities director.

As I proceeded I noticed that the living quarters for the seniors residing at this facility were located down long, wide hallways extending out from the hub area in a sun-burst fashion. I observed that these rooms were well furnished with full baths, accommodating one or two se- niors per room. As I viewed these hallways I couldn't help but notice that traffic was very intense with seniors, doctors, and staff coming and going.

I also noticed that the center was equipped with individual rooms for television and movie watching, lis- tening to music, reading and writing, attending classes, prayer groups, and for holding meetings. There was also

2

a large activity room, located between the hub area and the center's large dining room. It was staffed with an activities director and assistants who were given the task of scheduling a wide variety of activities for seniors on a daily basis. One of the main activities was bingo, the preferred choice of seniors.

In this activities room I met with and introduced myself to the activities director, and she in turn introduced herself and thanked me for volunteering. She then escorted me to the dining room, where a small group of seniors was anxiously waiting to play bingo. While walking to the dining room, I was told that I was the only one that had responded to the care center's newspaper ad for bingo volunteers. I was surprised to hear this, thinking that there would have been more volunteers than just me. I was anxious to get started, not knowing whether the seniors would feel comfortable with me as their caller.

My immediate reaction on entering the dining room was, Wow! A senior myself, I was about to call bingo for seniors. Of the ten seniors in attendance, nine were females, and only one was male. As I started calling bingo, with the activity director at my side, I could not help but notice that these seniors were confined to wheelchairs or needed walkers. I was surprised that a prize was only given to the winner of the last blackout game. That changed when I began calling bingo routinely, with prizes awarded to winners of each and every game played.

I realized early on that many prizes were needed, and I went about acquiring them through donations and by purchasing items at garage sales, etc.

Henry Nelson Feste

The main contributor of funds for purchasing prizes is my daughter. She and my wife have contributed much of their time and are the driving force behind my volunteer work. More to follow regarding the role prizes play in the game of bingo.

The activities staff notified seniors in their monthly newsletter that "Bingo with Mr. Henry" would be an ongoing event held at 3:00 p.m. on Wednesdays in the center's dining room. Seniors responded in increased numbers to thirty or more, most of them females, with just a few males. The activity staff thanked me for bringing this about, and they further said that, like me, they would now be awarding prizes to all winners on the days they called bingo. "Halleluiah!" was my response.

My granddaughter who lives nearby helped during the summer of 2009 and 2010, doing volunteer work to accumulate service hours for high school. She helped with the set-up and clean-up after bingo. As well, she brought the cart of prizes to the winners of each game. She also sat and helped those seniors play who had poor vision or hearing. Help also came from my out-of-state daughter and granddaughter while visiting from California during the summer of 2010.

Louise, one of the volunteers at the center, helped to set up and clean up after bingo. Occasionally she sat with seniors needing help. Her two preteen granddaughters volunteered during the summer of 2010. They too helped bring the cart of prizes to the winners and with cleaning up afterward. What a pleasure having them as helpers at such a young age. After a while Louise was not seen, and I heard that the reason for this was that she no longer volunteered at the center. I was sorry to hear this, knowing that I would miss her help and that of her granddaughters.

The prizes given out when I first started calling bingo were confined to Mardi Gras beads and trinkets donated by my wife and me and our daughters. We attended many Mardi Gras celebrations while living in New Orleans for thirty-eight years before we were forced to relocate to the Houston area after Hurricane Katrina's devastation in 2005. Once these carnival items were gone, stuffed animals, dolls, and beanie babies took their place as prizes. These were donated by my daughter's girls as well as bags of stuffed animals donated by neighbors, friends, and others, or purchases at garage sales and other venues. Once when we were running low on stuffed animals and beanie babies, a neighbor of mine saved the day by donating various new items such as picture frames, vases, wallets, pocket books, purses, porcelain pieces, dishware, glassware, wood ware, figurines, bracelets, costume jewelry, knick knacks, etc. The seniors were delighted with this variety of items to choose from, but they still preferred stuffed animals/dolls.

While prizes continue to be gained through donations, others come from purchases made at garage sales, flea markets, church consignment sales, supermarkets, big box stores, or at bargain stores such as the Salvation Army, Goodwill, and Dollar Tree. Stuffed animals are desired more than other items. The reason for this, I believe, is that the seniors are able to give them to their grandkids or great-grandkids, or they just keep them for themselves, turning back the clock to a childhood love of stuffed animals.

In the area where my wife and I live, there are several large community garage sales held each year at summer's end and in early fall. My wife and I attend these one-day events, collecting lots of items for use as bingo prizes. Items are purchased or given away by homeowners not wanting to keep them at the end of the garage sale. This is a prime source for stockpiling prizes as are yearly sales held by churches of various denominations. The numerous items collected at these events are sorted in our home, and only those in good condition are retained, while others are discarded. The acceptable items are then stored in one of our guest rooms. This room does fill up, but it also empties quickly as items are removed and awarded to bingo winners.

Girl Scout cookies were introduced in February 2011 for seniors to pick from the prizes offered at bingo, and they were popular enough that various brands of boxed cookies and bagged candy were added to the prize list. They are purchased at large supermarkets and box stores at discount prices. At least one or two of these treats are included for seniors who prefer them over other bingo prizes.

I'm told that it's not just bingo prizes that I give out, but also my personality, my congeniality, my camaraderie, and my humor that make "Bingo with Mr. Henry" so popular. Some have even said that it's because I'm a "senior hottie," and I do get that impression at times. I'm no Cary Grant or John Wayne, but I do notice some of the ladies gazing at me with a twinkle in their eye as I call bingo. While this may not be true—and probably isn't—but what matters is that "Bingo with Mr. Henry" brings them joy as they struggle with aging and mental and/or physical illnesses of all sorts. Playing bingo is a diversion and a moment of escape from all their woes. They play well up into their nineties and even one hundreds, until illness or mental issues take over and bingo is no longer possible.

On returning home from bingo, weighted down by my large square plastic bin of leftover prizes, I feel very tired and emotionally drained. My wife takes the bin of prizes from me, then inventories and stores them in our guest room. I drink a bottle of water first and then flop down in my favorite living room chair, feeling very tired. Thoughts of bingo swirl in my head as I try to rest. I get up and make notes of my thoughts before they fade or disappear. This routine has gone on for almost three years now, with the notes I have kept being the basis for my narrative up till now and hereafter.

At the outset, the center's seniors were told that I myself was a senior at age seventy-five and that they were my bingo pals. Further that bingo with me as their caller would be a fun thing, with lots of laughter, songs, prizes for winners, and with no silent library type of atmosphere allowed. On my first day, I held up a bingo card displaying the letters/numbers B1 thru O75 telling them that it represented my lifespan from childhood thru adulthood and stopping at age seventy-five. I joked that at age seventy-five I was still on the bingo chart, but not for long. I determined then, and later on, by a show of hands and by seniors admitting their age, that the vast majority of them were over seventy-five years of age and well into their eighties and nineties and a few reaching one hundred.

While calling bingo for almost three years now, I have been exposed to numerous seniors/caregivers of various personalities, attitudes, moods, and/or temperaments, and I have chosen some of them over others as interesting subjects, as revealed hereafter. I have given them fictitious names to conceal their true identities

Caregiver Marsha, at seventy-three, had cared for Minnie for twelve years. Minnie, at ninety-six, required constant care, and in September 2010 she passed away. Marsha lost someone very dear to her. Afterward Marsha faced serious health issues herself, but she has recovered and is back as a caregiver. She continues to attend bingo and help in any way she can. Her effervescent personality and feistiness livens up the games, to say the least. Bingo is not dull when she attends, and she has attended from the start of my calling bingo.

Beth, at sixty-six, is a caregiver for Heather and plays bingo for herself and Heather. She sat at the same table with Marsha and Minnie prior to Minnie's death. She's sweet, soft-spoken, considerate of others, and a pleasure to be around. She says she enjoys playing bingo with me as caller. She's very complimentary of my style of bingo, which she says brings enjoyment not just to her but to the other players. Lately Beth has not been playing bingo and is no longer the caregiver for Heather. I occasionally see her caring for another senior. Beth's husband used to play bingo while sitting beside her, and he followed her around while she performed her duties as a caregiver. Beth told me that she and her husband were childhood sweethearts, but sadly he now has Alzheimer's and requires constant care.

Gerry, caregiver for Amelia, also plays bingo. Amelia suffers with Alzheimer's and is confined to a wheelchair. Gerry carefully watches over her as they both play bingo. Amelia sleeps on and off during the games, and when she awakens she often yells out "Bingo!" startling other players and finding this humorous. Gerry's robust personality contributes to the overall fun of playing bingo. She also helps those seniors play who are unable to hear well or read numbers. And at times she has helped by pushing the cart of prizes around to winners.

Wally, using a walker and fitted with an oxygen tank, usually sits at Gerry's table, and she watches over him while he plays. Wally's walker is draped with all sorts of things, including an American flag signifying his patriotism. He likes bingo and is disappointed if he does not win. He's a sore loser in that he thinks that he should always win and he's not happy when he loses. When he does win, he picks candy or cookies as a prize, if available. Wally likes to remove prizes from the plastic bin I bring to bingo. Removing them, he then places them on the prize cart, and while doing so he continually comments in a loud, mumbling voice that's hard to understand. During the games he's constantly mumbling, but this is not a distraction, as the games go on without complaints. Wally illuminates the room with his presence, much to the delight of all those attending, including myself.

Henry Nelson Feste

There were two wheelchair players, Rita and Barbara, who attended bingo in the beginning. Rita, who had some sort of back problem, was bent over unable to sit up straight in her wheelchair. She spoke softly and was difficult to hear. That's probably why she sat very near to me, so she could be heard calling "BINGO!" Barbara was reliant upon an oxygen tank, with oxygen tubes protruding from her nose. She was polite and always thanked me for the pleasure she experienced playing bingo. She sat very quietly playing, never commenting or complaining. Not long after I started calling bingo, Rita and Barbara no longer showed up, and I was informed of the sad news that they had passed away.

The deaths of Rita and Barbara came as a shock, but there were more deaths to come and also seniors no longer able to play because of aging, bad health, or mental issues. It's the road's end for many here, and they are coping as best they can. Bingo helps them cope and brings a certain amount of pleasure to their lives.

Maggie, aged eighty-eight, besides being a very active bingo player, was a big help in passing out bingo cards and chips and collecting them after the games were over. She did this from the start of my calling bingo, but does so no longer as age has taken its toll. She used to walk on her own, except for occasionally needing a walker, but now she's fully reliant on the walker. Early on her daughter and daughter's husband attended bingo with her, but they have not been seen of late. Maggie is outgoing, very talkative, and effervescent. She brings her effervescence to the games, encouraging others to joke, laugh, sing, and have fun. Bingo is not to be played in silence, with the only sounds heard being winners yelling bingo and losers groaning. To avoid this, jokes, laughter, and even singing are encouraged, and Maggie's presence helps make this happen.

As I write this I no longer can count on her help since she only attends bingo sporadically. It's not because she no longer has the desire, but rather it's her memory that limits her activity. She has difficulty remembering what time and day of the week it is and often misses bingo for that reason, or she forgets that bingo is even being played. The last time she played she insisted that she is sixty-seven years old when actually she's eighty-eight. She looks much older than in the past, but still effervescent and still able to play and illuminate the room.

Marilyn, at eighty-three, was also a bingo regular and helped passing out bingo cards and chips when I first started calling bingo. She was able to walk on her own then, but now she is fully dependent on a wheelchair. Marilyn always gave me a big smile and a hug upon arriving to play bingo and also upon leaving. Sadly she began having mood swings, temper tantrums, and bad behavior that worsened over time, and she no longer plays. She now is under the nurses' close watch and care. She doesn't even recognize me anymore, when not so long ago she was full of smiles and hugs. She wears baseball caps, and sometimes she is seen in the hallways wearing the cap I gave her. Most of the time, though, she's confined to her room.

Thelma is a kind-hearted, extremely helpful person. At forty-seven, she is one of the younger players at bingo. She walks on her own without the aid of a walker or wheelchair and appears healthy, but she admits to having health issues. She helps those having vision or hearing problems play the game. She also helps setting up for bingo and cleaning up afterward. During bingo, she helps immensely by bringing the cart of bingo prizes to winners. Without her help I would have to push the cart myself, thus delaying the games. She's an intense bingo player who enjoys the game, and she likes winning. She tells me that she lives with her husband at the center, but he hardly ever leaves the room, due to health problems.

The activities staff praises Thelma for being very helpful to them throughout the day. But they have said that she has to be stopped from bringing the cart of bingo cards and chips into the dining room at 3:30 p.m. on Wednesdays while a karaoke player or musical group is entertaining the seniors. Music entertainment is offered once a month on Wednesdays from 2:30 to 3:30 p.m. This entertainment is supposed to end at exactly 3:30 p.m. so that bingo with Mr. Henry can begin. The problem arises when this musical entertainment goes beyond 3:30, which it usually does, and infringes on bingo. While the seniors enjoy the musical entertainment, they object to it infringing on bingo time, especially when it's bingo with Mr. Henry. I'm confronted by seniors when this happens with complaints about bingo being cut short. I must say that this is proof positive of seniors' love for the game of bingo over all else. They do enjoy musical entertainment so long as it doesn't interfere with bingo.

When I started, Timmy was the one and only male player, and he sat at a table with Maggie. She helped Timmy as he had difficulty reading bingo numbers. Timmy was an avid Elvis Presley fan, and when coaxed, he would sing part of an Elvis tune during bingo. On occasions I'd visit Timmy in his room, and he'd be watching an Elvis movie. I had toured Elvis's Graceland in Memphis with my wife, and I gave copies of the pictures we took to Timmy, along with a CD of Elvis hit tunes. He was delighted and especially liked the pictures of Graceland. He also was given a large pair of pink Mardi Gras beads that reminded him of Elvis's pink Cadillac.

Timmy failed to show up for bingo one week, and I was told that he was ill and had been transferred to the hospital. While he was expected to get better, he never did, and sadly he passed away, without my knowing or saying good-bye. I was fond of Timmy, and he of me, and I wondered whether family and friends were present to bid him farewell. Sadly I was not afforded that opportunity.

Meredith, at ninety six or ninety-seven—or so she said—was a very outspoken, feisty lady who made her presence loudly known at bingo. She was one of the regulars, and occasionally her daughter attended. She always spoke out during the games saying that she could not hear the numbers being called or that the numbers were being called too slow or too fast! She complained about bingo being too noisy, to the objection of others who liked it that way. She repeated bingo numbers out loud after I called them, much to the annoyance of others, and I had to put a stop to it. She often complained out loud that she was unlucky and never won, even as I reminded her of winning her fair share. When she did win, she often expressed dissatisfaction with the bingo prizes being offered, and she either refused or reluctantly accepted her prize.

One week she did not show up, and I was saddened to learn that she had passed away. She livened up bingo with her feistiness for sure. I never saw the daughter after her mom's passing to offer my condolences and to tell her how I enjoyed her mom's presence at bingo and the way she had livened up the games.

Beatrice was one of the regulars at the start of my calling bingo. She sat at my table, or one very nearby, so her soft, quivering voice could be heard when calling out the winning numbers. She trembled as she sat confined to a wheelchair playing bingo. She was always smiling and in good spirits, even as her health worsened as the weeks passed. Large black spots appeared on her face, and she appeared very weak the last time she played. Not seeing her anymore, I was told that she had passed away. I was saddened to hear this, and hopefully bingo brought her enjoyment at life's end. She was a lovely lady who enjoyed bingo to the very end. I still have visions of her at bingo to this very day.

Naomi was grumpy, like the Disney character Grumpy in *Snow White and the Seven Dwarves*. She always picked the same two bingo cards. Both small and large cards are used, but she refused to use the small cards. She only played with casino-type chips rather than the small orange plastic chips. Confined to a wheelchair, she was brought to bingo by her daughter or a nurse. Naomi yelled out if I was calling the numbers too slow or too fast. Whenever I called B-8, she'd yell, "I'd rather have a V8!" She began wearing an oxygen tank and slept during the games as her health deteriorated. She quit playing at 103 years of age, and not too long after that, she passed away. When I call B8 during bingo, I always yell "I'd rather have a V8," in remembrance of Naomi.

Eloise attended most of the time but never played bingo. She preferred sitting in her wheelchair at the back of the room waiting for the games to end. When they did, she wheeled herself up front and checked out the prizes left on the cart and picked one that she wanted. I told her that the prizes were just for bingo winners, but in the end I allowed her to have one. Not seeing her at bingo, I was shocked to learn that she had been found dead in her room, and further that her room was filled with stuffed animals/dolls from bingo. I was told that these items were given to the activities staff and were reused as prizes at bingo games other than mine.

If Eloise only knew, I wonder what her reaction would have been to her stuffed animals/dolls being re-used as bingo prizes. She probably would have reacted by admitting that, for the most part, they were given to her at my bingo. Hey! I'm glad that the activities staff got to use them, and I'm sure Eloise would have agreed.

Sarah sits silently in her wheelchair in the back of the dining room. Like Eloise, she does not want to play bingo, just watch. Attempts at getting her to play by putting cards and chips on the table in front of her or by having a volunteer help her have failed. As soon as bingo ends, she wheels herself up to the prize cart and points to a prize she likes. She cannot speak, so she uses sign language to plead for a certain prize. Needless to say, I give her the prize she wants, as I did with Eloise. There

15

are times when other seniors complain about my giving her a prize she did not win, but that has not stopped me from doing so, for I believe it would not be understood by Sarah or be fair to her, in her situation.

Molly plays bingo regularly and, contrary to others, says that it's considerate of me to give Sarah a prize she did not win. Further, she says her room is across the hall from Sarah's, and she's awakened quite often by Sarah crying. Molly insists that Sarah cries throughout the night, every night. I say to Molly, how can this be since Sarah cannot speak? I have noticed, however, that she's often asleep in her wheelchair, waiting to collect her bingo gift when bingo ends. I often have to awaken her, and I wonder if this could be sleep deprivation brought about by Sarah crying during the night?

Dora is a warm-hearted, avid bingo player. Dora has been dubbed Doris Day, past star of movies and television. When Dora wins, everyone sings "Que Sera Sera," a song made popular by Doris Day starring in the 1956 movie *The Man Who Knew Too Much*, an oldie-but-goodie movie. She's cheerful and smiles often during the games and is very serious about winning. With her hearing problem, she strains to hear the numbers called, and sometimes I have to repeat them for her. She goes out of her way to greet me when arriving for bingo and thanking me afterward. She's confined to a wheelchair, but she is able to maneuver around by herself without assistance. She enjoys winning at bingo and likens it to winning at the casino, only on a much smaller scale. She's been absent from bingo at times due to illness, and of late she does not appear to have the stamina she once had, but she still plays and enjoys the game.

Karen, one of the younger players at fifty-three, had a large cast around her chest, which was removed, but she remained confined to a wheelchair, still unable to walk. The reason for the cast was that she had broken her back. Ouch! She always smiles and has a good personality. If one of the seniors needs help hearing or reading numbers called, she does not hesitate to help. She has helped when I've mispronounced a senior's name by whispering the correct pronunciation in my ear. She smokes cigarettes outdoors, as smoking is prohibited in the center. I told her that smoking is a bad habit, but this has not stopped her from smoking.

Just after bingo one Wednesday, she informed me that she was being transferred out of state to another care center. She said that beside her back problem, she had other health issues. She cried big tears and hugged me, saying how much she would miss the fun she had playing bingo. I often wonder how Karen is doing now, whether her health has deteriorated or improved, and if she still plays bingo.

Karen sat at the same table with Tina and her mother, along with three other ladies, all confined to wheelchairs. This table was crowded with lots of conversation and laughter during the games. Tina was not a resident, but her mother was. Her mother, Samantha, is ninety-two and loved winning stuffed animals that she held very close to her. This group played every week, until Karen left the center and Tina took ill and stopped attending. A relative did attend once and played bingo with Tina's mom, Samantha. This relative told me that Tina had cancer and was at home recovering and was expected to return. After months of recovery, Tina did return with her mom, and I welcomed them back. As luck would have it, Tina's mom won the final blackout game, and she was overjoyed at receiving the prize of a large stuffed pink bunny that she held close to her. Tina, battling cancer, still cares dearly for her mom, and God bless her for that.

Beth, upon entering the room, will approach the cart of prizes and say out loud, "What kind of goodies do you have for us this week?" She speaks out during the games and joins in the sing-alongs and especially likes singing "Que Sera Sera." I once asked her how old she was, but when I guessed eighty-three, she laughed, saying she was much older at ninety-four. She calls herself the "Energizer Bunny" that just keeps going and going. What an amazing woman, young at heart and so energized at ninety-four. Her daughters visit her often and play bingo along with her. Beth says her husband passed away years ago, at age sixty-seven.

Jill, at seventy-three, regularly plays bingo. She's confined to a wheelchair with a brace on her leg, and she occasionally wears an oxygen tank as she suffers with asthma and emphysema. She plays bingo with a vengeance, determined to win, and appears disappointed when she doesn't. Her husband and daughters have attended on a number of occasions. One of her daughters has donated jewelry to give out as prizes. Jill is kind and considerate, wanting others to enjoy the games just as much as she does. She sat at the same table across from Annie before Annie passed away.

Jill and Annie, at ninety-five, were close friends. Annie appeared very reserved and alert for her age, sitting in her wheelchair. She seemed to enjoy bingo. On occasion her son visited her during bingo, and he would say to me that I was the featured attraction at bingo, bringing joy to all the players. After a while, Annie no longer attended bingo, and Jill told me that Annie was extremely depressed, refused to eat, and did not want to live anymore. Annie did get her wish and passed away. It's always shocking to hear of the death of a person you come to know, and I wondered how Annie's son took the news of his mother's passing.

Joan, at ninety-one and confined to a wheelchair, is another one of the regulars. She is very alert for her age and does not hesitate to speak her mind about jokes, songs sung, or comments made during bingo. Her comments help to liven up the games. Joan enjoys bingo, and she likes winning. She's always smiling and in good spirits. She enjoys my bingo calling—or so she has said many times. She recently celebrated her seventy-eighth anniversary, her husband having passed away years ago. She has children, and she boasts of having many grandchildren and great-grandchildren. Several of her sons come to visit her on occasion. She's petite and has gray hair and boasts of having had red hair when she was younger. She has arthritis and no longer plays the piano, due to the pain experienced in her hands. She says she's played the piano practically all her life until arthritis took away the joy of it. Joan turned ninety-two on her birthday in September 2011, and we all sang happy birthday to her. What an amazing lady, still very alert at ninety-two years of age and still liking bingo.

Henry Nelson Feste

Ronda is solely reliant upon a wheelchair, like most others at the center, and she sits at the same table with Joan. They sit in their wheelchairs across from each another. Ronda is a very lucky bingo player, winning most often. The rules are that you can only win one game, except for the last two games that everyone is eligible to win. Ronda, on one occasion, won a regular game as well as the final two games, winning the special prizes set aside for the last two games. "Ronda the lucky one!" is what we all call her. Ronda likes it when I sing excerpts from songs made popular by Dean Martin during bingo. She tells me that these lyrics remind her of once meeting him, years ago, at a celebrity golf tournament. To this day, she has vivid memories of Dino and how handsome he was.

Bernice, at ninety-seven, was part of a small group of players attending when I first started calling bingo. She liked sitting in her wheelchair by herself at a table in the back of the dining room. I believe this was the table she was assigned to for meals. She's petite and speaks softly, so she was hardly heard when yelling out "Bingo!" She played bingo for a good while, before physical and mental issues put a stop to it. The last time she played was during the summer of 2010, when my granddaughter sat and helped her play. She's still at the center, but her bingo days are over. She occasionally wheels herself into the bingo room and disrupts the games and often has to be removed before bingo can be resumed.

Rebecca, one of the assistant activity directors, has her mother, Jamie, ninety-four, residing at the center. Jamie played bingo on occasions up until lately when age issues prevented her from playing anymore. Rebecca still brings her mom to bingo to watch, but she often falls asleep in her wheelchair in the back of the room. When she played bingo she always came up to my table afterward to tell me how much she enjoyed herself, and she thanked me for the pleasure I brought her calling bingo. Her poetic comment, said to me on one occasion, will always be remembered: "When all of us are playing bingo in heaven, Saint Peter will have you, Henry, as our caller."

"Suzie come lately" she's called after the old saying "Johnny come lately" in that she always arrives late to bingo. She walks into the room aided by her walker and interrupts my calling bingo, asking if bingo is over. I say no, of course, and tell her to pick up bingo cards and chips to play at the start of the next game. She prefers sitting by herself at a table, and she wins her fair share of games. She picks a stuffed animal when she does win. Sometimes during play, she starts coughing and yelling loudly that her nose is running. When this happens one of the players hands her some Kleenex to blow her nose, and bingo resumes. Suzie's explanation for coming late to bingo is that she's somewhat of a loner and does not like mingling with others before bingo starts.

I cringe when Donna wins because she has to go through the whole cart of prizes before she decides on the one she wants. The next game cannot start until she picks a prize, and the delay frustrates the rest of the players, who want to play as many games as possible within the time frame allotted. I try to tell her to hurry up and pick her prize, but that doesn't work, and to make matters worse, she's usually not satisfied with the prize she picks. As soon as bingo ends, she often comes up to the bingo cart and returns the prize she won for one of the leftover prizes. The dictionary should have a picture of Donna under the definition of undecided.

Only occasionally does Emma show up for bingo, and she's assisted by a nurse when she does. She sits alone at a table with her walker nearby. She sits staring into the distance, ignoring the bingo cards and chips left for her by the nurse. After a while she stands up with the aid of her walker and slowly walks around talking to herself, seemingly confused and lost. The first time this happened several of the attending seniors said that this was typical of her and that she needed a nurse's help. Bingo is usually delayed until she's removed by an activities staff member.

Serena, at eighty-four, uses a walker, and occasionally her daughter Donna plays bingo with her. They sit at a table close to mine. Serena enjoys my style of bingo and does not hesitate to express her dissatisfaction when entertainers perform past 3:30 p.m. and infringe on the time allotted for bingo. Serena, like others, enjoys the entertainers—as long as they leave within the time frame allotted for them. Serena always chooses jewelry for a prize when available, or stuffed animals for one of her grandkids or great-grandkids. She has four grown children, and her husband passed away about seventeen years ago, she says.

The table where I call bingo is in the front of the dining room. I stand for about one hour and a half during bingo, calling sixteen or more games every Wednesday.

Thus far twenty games are the most ever called. Bingo starts at 3:00 or 3:30 p.m. and ends at around 4:45 p.m. Seniors sit at tables during bingo playing with two cards, except for the last blackout game, which is restricted to one card.

There are seniors that sit in the back of the room as onlookers. Before bingo starts, the seniors gather around the cart of prizes and decide on the special prizes to be awarded for the last two games, namely the game before blackout and the final blackout game. A show of hands decides which prize is to be awarded for each game. Excitement builds during the blackout game when it comes down to players only needing one or two numbers to win. They all want to win at blackout and receive the special prize.

There are usually three players at my table: Cindy to my left, Evelyn to my right, and Roger across from me, although recently Roger has moved to another table and plays less often. Cindy, at sixty-three, is confined to a wheelchair. She's very quiet and soft-spoken. She likes sitting at my table so that her soft, whispering voice can be heard as she calls out "Bingo!" and her winning numbers. She is very pleasant and likeable. She doesn't miss bingo, except when she's ill. One of these illnesses was contagious, keeping her under confinement with a face mask and away from bingo until she was completely cured. She leaves immediately after bingo ends and arrives very early to secure a seat at my table. Lately she's been melancholy, and when I questioned her about this, she shrugged her shoulders in reply.

Henry Nelson Feste

Evelyn was ninety-eight when I first started calling bingo. She's confined to a wheelchair with one amputated leg, arthritis, and various other age-related illnesses. She needs help getting around in her wheelchair, and on several occasions I wheeled her from the dining room down the hallway to her room. Along the way, I observed that nurses were feeding or caring for ill seniors in wheelchairs, on gurneys, or bedridden in their rooms. This scene was unsettling to me, as it must be for seniors not requiring this kind of intensive care and having to witness this on a daily basis.

Evelyn's very sweet and everyone loves her. She is very positive, never complains, and loves playing bingo, especially with me as caller—so she says. She's very special to me. She wishes that the games would never end, and she hardly ever misses bingo. Evelyn lived in Louisiana, where she was a school teacher for many years. She is now a centurion having recently turned one hundred with an elaborate birthday party celebrated at the care center. All of the care center's administrative staff, nurses, and residents attended, as did I and some of Evelyn's family members.

Recently Evelyn has begun to forget to clear her card after each game and has to be reminded to do so. And sometimes she fails to place chips on her card over numbers called. As a centurion, this is excusable, and it's good that I'm close by to help. Amazing though, that at one hundred-plus she's still very active and able to play and enjoy the game of bingo.

Just recently Cindy's place at my table, across from Evelyn, was occupied by Darlene, in that Cindy arrived late and had to sit somewhere else. Darlene is somewhat caustic and outspoken and began bothering Evelyn, criticizing her for not immediately clearing her card before the start of a new game. I could see that this was upsetting Evelyn, and accordingly I reprimanded Darlene, telling her she would be moved to another table if she did not stop. This put an end to it, with Darlene remaining quiet up to the end of bingo. But she still presented a problem in that she played with two instead of one bingo card for the final blackout game. She refused to give up one of the cards saying that she had paid for it. Thankfully she did not win blackout, as I would have had to disqualify her.

Roger, at fifty-eight, confined to a wheelchair with a brace on one leg, sat across the way from me until recently, when he moved to another table. He is one of just a few male players. His speech is impaired, and he needs help calling out numbers when he wins. He's helpful in that he keeps track of the number of games played, as I tend to forget. He's very polite and considerate of others playing the game. He has a keen eye for the nurses and gives some of his bingo prizes to them as well as others.

She's *The Thief of Bagdad* from the classic old 1940s movie, as I have dubbed her. She's been caught more than once at thievery, stealing prizes from the bingo prize cart. When confronted she has apologized and given back the items stolen. She continues to play and is closely watched. There's another bingo player with the same tendencies who is also closely watched. Can it be that the cart of bingo prizes is too tempting for some to resist?

Martha is not a resident but rather the wife of John who is a resident at the center. Martha cares for John with Alzheimer's and other health issues. She wheels him, lying prostrate or propped up on a mobile bed, into the room, placing him and herself at a table to play bingo. They are newcomers, and Martha plays, but not John, who sleeps most of the time or stares into the distance when awake. Martha's truly devoted, spending six hours every day at the center caring for John. She said that on one occasion John was found in his room one morning sleeping on the floor. At bingo recently with Martha, John, and their daughter Marilyn attending, I sang a few lines from an Elvis Presley hit song, then stopped to ask who made the song popular, and everyone roared "Elvis!" Since I knew just a few of the lines, Marilyn took over and sang the whole song beautifully to cheers at the end.

A unique prize that the seniors liked, as did some of the nurses and activities staff members, was donated by a friend and neighbor of mine. On one of his trips to New Orleans he brought back several dozen large syrup-flavored popcorn balls each wrapped in clear plastic. He told me that these were very delicious, homemade Louisiana-style popcorn balls. My friend knew that I called bingo for seniors, and he handed over these popcorn balls for them to enjoy. Sure enough, they were enjoyed by seniors and nurses having Louisiana roots. A party atmosphere prevailed as seniors, nurses, and members of the activities staff sat around the bingo tables eating popcorn balls.

There are numerous nurses/assistant nurses at this care center, and often they provide assistance and/or medicine to seniors as they play bingo. Sometimes they require seniors to be removed immediately for treatment. Some seniors go reluctantly, while others refuse and resist but eventually do leave. One of these nurses is named Brenda, and she told me that her hobby is collecting monkeys, and so whenever I come across stuffed, porcelain, or brass monkeys in my search for bingo prizes, I give them to her, and she's most appreciative.

There are seniors in wheelchairs that obviously have behavioral problems, and occasionally they wheel themselves unescorted into the dining room when bingo is in progress. When they do, they usually bump into the wheelchairs of players, annoying them and interrupting bingo. Nurses or activities staff personnel have to remove them, sometimes forcibly, so that bingo can resume. One female wheeled in behind me once while I was calling bingo numbers and grabbed hold of my back pocket and refused to let go. While nurses were pulling her wheelchair backward they were pulling me along with her, as she held tightly onto my back pocket. Noticing this, the nurses stopped and forcibly removed her hand from my pocket and wheeled her from the room. Another female wheeled herself into the room, bumping into wheelchairs as she pulled seniors' arms and removed bingo cards and chips from tables. And on other occasions, seniors have come in and stuffed orange-colored bingo chips into their mouths, thinking they were candy.

Then there are the seniors battling dementia or other mental disorders that quietly enter the room and wheel about with expressionless looks on their faces. They are docile, causing no problem other than occasionally bumping into wheelchair-confined players or blocking

27

the aisles between tables. One such person likes sitting quietly in her wheelchair, staring at me while I'm calling bingo. Can this be because I'm a senior hottie? I don't think so, but then again maybe.

Sometimes deranged wheelchair seniors are brought by nurses into the room and given bingo cards and chips in hopes that they will play. In most instances they do not, and instead they interrupt the games by talking nonsensically to themselves or by grabbing cards and chips from players or by standing up, activating their loud wheelchair alarms. One such incident happened when a nurse pushed an unruly senior in a wheelchair into the room, positioned her at a table to play bingo, and left the room. This senior then wheeled herself away from the table and roamed around the room speaking nonsense to the seniors at other tables, who ignored her, wanting to be left alone. Bingo had to be delayed until a member of the activities staff removed her.

I call them the "beep seniors," those who sit quietly in their wheelchairs staring into the distance until they stand up, setting off their wheelchair alarm, giving off a continuous, loud, beep-like sound until they sit down. The problem is that they don't sit down on their own and require the know-how of a nurse to set them down and remove them from the room. Bingo is on hold until all of this is ironed out, and the irony of it is that they were deliberately put there even though they were neither interested nor capable of playing bingo.

Seniors cope with all of the above disturbances and more while playing bingo, and they just go on playing. Bingo is their passion, and they are not about to let anything interfere with it. Most of the time bingo is played smoothly, yet interruptions of the kind I have mentioned do occur quite often.

Newcomers regularly show up for bingo, along with their varied personalities, likes, and dislikes. They join what I call the regulars of old, who have attended ever since the beginning of my calling bingo almost three years ago. Sadly, these old regulars are less in number, and I'm seeing more newcomers in their place. As this happens I'm concerned that newcomers won't come to know and like my style of bingo as much as the remaining old guard regulars have. I have noticed that, contrary to the original group of regulars, the newcomers seem to be more docile, less apt to speak out, joke, laugh, or sing during bingo. This is not my kind of bingo, and I'm hoping that in due course this will change, or the situation will be helped with an influx of feisty newcomers.

I work closely with the activities staff at the care center, and in my view, they work very hard and effortlessly, affording seniors a variety of activities to enjoy. Also, the health/therapy care afforded seniors at this facility via its staff, doctors, nurses, caregivers, volunteers, etc. appears to be of very high quality.

In my further view, there is room for improvement in preventing deranged seniors from intruding upon and disrupting bingo, as has happened and as I have witnessed and discussed at length above. This may be difficult to accomplish, but it's certainly worth the effort toward improving bingo at this care center.

My story ends here, and I hope that it's been as enlightening for you as the reader as it has been for me to tell. As I write this, I believe I may stop calling bingo on my seventy-eighth birthday, a few months from now. Then again, only God knows what the future holds, and for me, it may be to continue calling bingo for seniors. Bingo, the game loved by children and adults alike, and especially seniors. I'm sure my "Bingo Pals" would want "Bingo with Mr. Henry" to carry on forever.

THE END